Spirit Dogs

poiêsis press

Spirit Dogs

How to Be Your Dog's Personal Shaman

Jane Galer

poiêsis press
Mendocino   Manasota Key

Poiêsis Press
An imprint of Poiêsis Publishing Group
Mendocino, California
poiesispress.com

©2016 by Jane Galer. All rights reserved.

Printed in the United States.
22 21 20 19 18 17 16   1 2 3 4 5

The author retains sole responsibility for the content of this book and asserts her moral, artistic, and intellectual rights of protection.

The content of this book is not a substitute for veterinary medicine. It is intended for the personal use of the dog/pet owner. It is not recommended nor wise to practice these exercises on any pet other than your own. The author is not responsible for actions, consequences, or outcomes that might occur as a result of following the methods and guidance in this book. Shamanic techniques should be recognized as powerful work and should never be attempted without respect and care.

ISBN 978-0-9981323-0-3

All illustrations: ©2016 by Kim Englishbee

All rights reserved. Beyond personal use, no part of this book may be used or reproduced by any means, graphic, electronic, or mechanical, including photocopying, recording, taping or by any information storage retrieval system without the written permission of the publisher except in the case of brief quotations embodied in critical articles and reviews. Individuals may reproduce end log pages for their own use only.

About Poiêsis Press:
Poiêsis \'poi-ah-sis\ n. Greek; a creation, beginning, the root word for poetry, as in a bringing forth

We view the creative process as the complicity between the energies of muse and of mind. It is this commingling of energy that we think of as poiêsis. Poiêsis Press is dedicated to care-taking the energy of artistic creation, not feeding from it. We seek by what we publish to understand the complicated intercourse of word and art: the distillation of the creative urge into ink on paper.

Printed on acid free paper.

Contents

Preface
    How Wolves Became Dogs   1

Introduction
    How to Be Your Dog's Personal Shaman   5

Chapter 1
    What Is a Shaman?   10

Chapter 2
    Energy Field Basics   18

Chapter 3
    The Pendulum   32

Chapter 4
    Tuning the Out of Balance Chakra   42

Chapter 5
    Decoupling Fight or Flight   47

Chapter 6
    Saying Goodbye   54

Final Words   60

Appendices
    What about cats, horses, & absentee animals?   64
    Making Your Own Pendulum   67
    Log Book   70

Jane's Dog Biscotti recipe   80

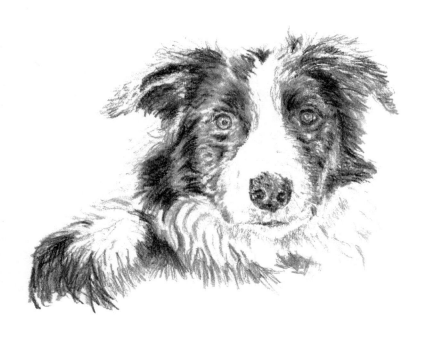

Preface

How Wolves Became Dogs

I like to imagine that the moment of first peaceful contact between wolf and man was something like this:

The women and children gathered nightly around the fire, for warmth, for cooking their daily catch of meat or fish, to sit and spin fibers, sew hides, shell nuts, and for the solace of the family group coming together after a long day of gathering, ranging far out into the hills or along the ocean strand in search of food. The men might have gone farther afield, gone for several days or even weeks as they followed a herd, tracking a big animal whose death would provide for the whole group for months. This fireside time was a time of storytelling and teaching. A time when the little ones nursed at their mother's breasts, and soon slept while the grandmother of the tribe told tales of the ancient ones. Perhaps one moonlit night they sat around the fire and one of their company stepped away from the light and chatter to seek the privacy of the bush and in doing so she came upon a young wolf. They stared at each other, startled, the wolf flat on his belly, immobile, eyes watching her every move, his body tense, but submissive. She was frightened at first, but soon saw that this wolf was starving, and his paw was lame and bloodied. Instead of responding as she had been taught and calling for help, the girl returned to the fire and took her bowl of food and softly stole away again into the dimness of the bush, back to the waiting wolf. She put the bowl down slowly before him and then sat back on her haunches and watched as he ate. When he finished, he seemed to relax, he shifted his gaze away from the wary apprehension of before, and pushed his body weight over to stretch out. His front legs stretching nearly to touch her own, and he looked at her as if asking for something more. But when she reached to touch his injured paw he rumbled a soft growl, so she knew she must wait.

How Wolves Became Dogs

The girl sat with the wolf as the night sky came over them, and even though she was tired and wanted her warm bed, she stayed with the wolf through the night, falling asleep only as dawn crept over the ridgeline. When she woke the wolf was gone.

Every night following the girl stole away from the campfire with her food and found the wolf waiting. At last he allowed her to touch him, first his good paw, then his injured one. She cleaned his wound, and fed him. And during the day when she was at her chores she worried about him. Weeks went by, and then the grandmother of the clan decided they would move their camp. The girl packed her things: her digging stick and her fur bedroll, her cup and bowl, and all the while she worried about her wolf. But she needn't have. As they walked away from their camp she saw behind her came the wolf trotting sure-footed and confident. The girl announced his presence to the others and quickly calmed their reaction of fear as the wolf sat quietly beside her, and it seemed to them as they gathered around that the wolf smiled. She explained how she'd found him; and the grandmother of the clan nodded, knowing all along that this was so, that this was to be. The grandmother explained that this meant the wolf would be their clan guardian, and that from now on, they would be the people of the Wolf.

The history of dogs' importance in the life of humans extends into the time before our remembering. Our attraction to, our dependence on, and our healing from our connection to dogs is deep in our genetics now. We understand them, and they understand us. Wolf as an archetype teaches us about tribal cooperation, teaching and hierarchy. About loyalty. Dog as an archetype teaches us about dedication, love, empathy, and... again....loyalty. There is a requirement, a pact, between our species as deep and open as our own hearts.

Introduction

How to Be Your Dog's Personal Shaman

Halfway through my training in shamanic energy medicine I was volunteering to perform sessions in energy healing with anyone who would sit still. Every time I worked on someone, my own skills improved and I understood the process better and better. One summer day I was at the lake house of my cousins. I hadn't seen them in years. I was driving across country to sort out my late father's effects and stopped in for some much needed TLC, the kind only family can provide. Pretty soon I was spreading out my medicine bundle on the bedroom floor and, one by one, giving energy medicine sessions to them. After the first two, hour and a half long sessions, we took a break, and I walked into the living room, leaving my medicine bundle open in the

Spirit Dogs

other room. We were laughing and talking in the living room when suddenly we realized the resident dog, a young tan and white hound mix named Scooter, was standing at the bedroom door: hair on end in a ridge down his back, growling, one of those tentative growls that says "I don't know what's out there and I'm not sure I should be growling at it, but this is my starting point." Scooter was growling at my *mesa*, my medicine bundle. I walked past Scooter into the bedroom and sat down next to my spread of tools—stones, rattles, incense, feathers—and spoke to Scooter, telling him it was OK, there was nothing to worry about here. Immediately he left the doorway and came into the room, sniffed the stones, pushed one particular stone with his nose, and then lay down across the whole lot! "Oh, me next!" he seemed to be saying. Scooter's family stood in the bedroom doorway, mouths gaping. I don't think they took me seriously with this shaman stuff until that moment. But the message was clear: if the dog thought it was a good idea, everyone else was on board.

How to Be Your Dog's Personal Shaman

Right from the start in my training I knew I wanted to use shamanic work with animals as well as people. It seemed so obvious. Every chance I had with my teachers I shifted the focus to how to apply what we were learning to dogs and cats. I wasn't the only one interested in this aspect of the work. In my first class I met one of our teachers, Christine Paul, who invited me to spend lunch time doing an energy healing on her dog, Tavi. Tavi was gravely ill with cancer, a tumor over one eye. It was an amazing and emotional hour watching Christine work with her dog, and seeing how calm and open Tavi was to the process. I was convinced that this was an important part of my own shamanic work. And Tavi kindly gave me an accepting kind of grace, allowing me to help ease her struggle. Our class had two veterinarians who were also there to learn the shamanic healing work. While it seems generally accepted that animals can help heal people—dogs, horses, cats—there's an undeniable healing connection, we don't often think of it in the other direction. We do our best to understand our individual pets, we take them to the vet when they're sick, we accept them

Spirit Dogs

---

into our families and take their love and loyalty. But there are times we wish we had answers. We adopt rescue dogs and wonder if the poor guy knows he's safe now. We think there's something wrong but we don't see any obvious physical symptoms, or toward the end of life, we wonder if they are ready for us to let them go. We have a lot of choices for seeking external help, including specialized trainers and veterinary professionals, and of course we would always do this for regular check ups, vaccinations, and serious and tenacious physical issues. But, wouldn't we all like to have a system we can use ourselves to take the energetic, emotional temperature of our beloved pets any time we wanted to? That's what this book is about.

In this book you will learn simple ways to check the energetic health of your dog. While my focus here is dogs for the sake of simplicity, these same techniques work on cats—really they will work on any warm-blooded pet. You will learn what shamanic energy medicine is, how the energy system of the body works, how checking in with your dog's energy field will benefit their health and socialization, and how to help your dog in an emergency. You don't need four years of shamanic lineage training to do this work with your dog. The techniques I will teach you here are simple and straightforward. The purpose is for you to establish a way to tune in to your dog's emotional energy on a day to day basis.

Caution: Energy medicine is strong and effective work. Without serious experience and training I do not recommend working on any animal except your own dog. This book is intended to increase the existing relationship you have with your own pet.

Chapter 1

What Is a Shaman?

Shamanism is not a religion. It's a system, a process, centered on the ability of certain individuals to access the many levels of consciousness in order to translate the needs and meanings of the universe for the community's well-being. The shaman is the go-between for Earth and her creatures, the one who directs our energy toward synchronicity and away from chaos. While often in primitive cultures the shaman is also the spiritual/religious priestly figure, the shaman in the modern world may walk all manner of religious preferences and still practice the same shamanic techniques and principles. My teachers, the Q'ero of Peru, are Catholic, but that religious preference is not relevant to, does not supersede nor drive, the shamanic

What Is a Shaman?

beliefs, rituals, or energy healing work that they hold. Shamanic techniques are, at their core, the same worldwide. Whether they are techniques of modern Western individuals or tribal shaman from indigenous cultures—from the Aboriginal Dreamtime, from Mongolia, Africa, Siberia, North America, the Celtic lands, Amazonia, or the Andes—the core theories are the same. To do the work you are going to learn, you don't need to become shaman. Becoming a shaman takes dedication, years of training, and something of a calling. But it will be useful to understand what principles underlie shamanic work.

First, the shaman uses a variety of techniques to access what I like to call the *superconscious*. No matter what time period we look at or what part of the world, the shaman use the same basic principles of expanded consciousness journeying. The point of the shamanic journey is to gain knowledge of the universe through a meditative state in order to benefit their community. The shaman uses a system of archetypal metaphor—whatever is meaningful to his own community, region, and locale. For example, the indigenous Sibe-

Spirit Dogs

rian shaman's most important role historically was as intermediary: speaking with the animal spirits in order to track game for hunters. Reindeer and Bear were significant allies as spirits. The Siberian shaman uses drumming to push her thinking brain aside and make room for the universe to speak. The drum is a meditative device, its resonant and repetitive sound facilitates the shamanic journey. Amazonian shaman use plant medicine to hasten the process by which they access the plant world for healing cures, they don't use drums because their climate isn't very friendly to building and maintaining drums, but they do use their own songs or whistling. Modern Western shaman with all possible tools available pick their preferred method—mine is whistling—and use that to create the altered state which allows them to track trauma lines: perhaps in order to soothe PTSD or restore equilibrium, identify past problems, and prepare the body for healing present issues. *Tracking*, as we call it, is the way the shaman uses the journey to give the body an energetic check up. Tracking involves the superconscious part of our brains. I like to describe it as

What Is a Shaman?

stepping out of the way of our thinking brains so that the real work of the universe can move forward. The shaman uses a variety of techniques to achieve this superconscious state from which he can then track a whole community or just one person. We're going to learn a simple tracking technique to use with our dogs which focuses on assessing the energetic health of the *chakras* of the body. We'll examine and define just what this means but basically we will learn to gauge the energetic body's well-being and in doing so we too will be accessing a small part of the superconscious energy that the shaman works with.

Let's stop for a moment and talk further about archetypal metaphor. Every culture has its mythology, its own collective personal story. In each culture, important structure is developed in order to secure community behavior that is in keeping with the rules of the village. It would be hard to find a culture, for example, that didn't have an archetypal "boogie man." Why? Because it's important to keep children in their beds and not have them wandering around the forest at night. Modern Western culture is developing and

Spirit Dogs

embellishing these archetypes as mythology all the time: that's the primary function of a good children's bedtime story. Think about your favorite childhood story and figure out who the archetypal characters are and what they stand for. Bilbo Baggins? Peter Pan? Mary Poppins? What are the lessons each of these characters teach us? Always carry an umbrella (sword, staff)? Well, maybe not, but attitude is everything and optimism will usually carry us through even the hardest challenge. Peter Pan? Magic has its place, everyone needs to use their imagination. My favorite Peter Pan character is obviously Nana. She's the dog! She's the family caregiver, the worrier, the protector, the ultimate in soft warm fuzzies. If I were going to do shamanic work on Nana, I would bet I'd find her heart chakra working hard but also that she's often afraid for the children in her care—she over-worries. I could ease some of that fear, not all of it, since that would mess with what Nana's job is in the family, but I can give her reassurance and lower her stress level. This is what you will learn to do using the tools of shamanic tracking taught in this book.

What Is a Shaman?

The shaman works in the realm of archetypes. Often, the shaman uses animal *familiars*—totem animal spirits—the essential creature, the archetype of the animal: Jaguar with a capital J that embodies all of the characteristics of the jaguar: predator, no known enemies, fearlessness, night work, etc. So for example, bears, owls, eagles, ravens, and coyotes, we pretty much instantly recognize the archetype of each of these animals. Often it seems we are drawn to a single animal, even if we've never seen one in the wild. The animal's spirit essence, or archetype, means something to us in a personal way. Working with the help of the animals as archetypes makes the shamanic journey more meaningful, easier, and also helps the shaman translate what he knows into language that his community can use successfully. The shaman uses the animal spirit's archetypal information as a metaphor to help explain to his community how to survive in the best possible way. We can see that the shaman acts as a go-between, representing the community as a whole or individuals within the community at the greater level of the universe. For our work with dogs,

Spirit Dogs

we want to access the archetype Dog, that perfect dog-ness, and bring that down into our own dog's energy field.

The shaman's *mesa* or medicine bundle is a collection of ritual tools often wrapped in a special cloth or tucked into a ritually important bag. In my mesa are a number of Zuni stone animal fetishes that I use when I work on clients. My favorite fetish is a black dog. This is dog with a capital D, the archetypal Dog. I've been a cat owner and a dog owner and a cat and dog at the same time owner, but lately we have dogs and particularly I have come to use my shamanic training more on dogs than other pets simply because that's what I've got. We are crazy about border collies. In our lives now are Tweed and Cavendish. Different as night and day but born of the same litter, purebred Scottish bloodline border collies. Cavendish is as healthy as a horse and eats like one. He's friendly but cautious and because he is nearly all black you wouldn't be sure he was a border collie except for the white at the end of his tail. Tweed is the alpha dog. He's energetic, devoted, and he has problems. Tweed has "collie nose," a form

What Is a Shaman?

of lupus called discoid lupus, which makes his nose scab and peel. He also has epilepsy. It is his grand mal seizures that brought me to writing this book. After his first seizure I took up my pendulum and checked his chakras. Everything was fine until I got to his head: the pendulum started bouncing and jerking, his 6th and 7th chakras were erratic and completely messed up. Well, of course they were! He'd just had a seizure! We comforted him, watched over him, helped him back to consciousness as loving companions should, but I also spent some time once he was safe and calm realigning those 6th and 7th aspects of his energetic being. This is what we're going to learn in this book: how to check your dog's chakras using a pendulum, and then what to do with the information gleaned from that tracking process.

The key to the work we are going to do here is that there exists a level of consciousness that is representative of our individual energy fields which any of us can access using a few simple techniques, and in doing so we can better communicate with each other and with our pets. Let's get started.

Chapter 2

Energy Field Basics

Each of us has an energy field. Think of it as an extension of your corporeal self. It surrounds your flesh and bone body and extends some distance out. That distance varies and depends on how your brain has decided to integrate your body with your energy field. I think it's possible that a small part of this field distance or size has to do with cultural influences. If you live in a culture that doesn't encourage personal space, where people tend to crowd on top of each other, or have experienced this while traveling, you'll know that sensation of someone being too close even if they aren't touching you. Sometimes the brain messes up the signals. Scientists have proposed that this might be a key to anorexia. The brain misreads

Energy Field Basics

---

where the body ends and sends the misinformation that the person is fat when they actually aren't. The brain might be reading the energetic body as corporeal. The energy field or energetic body is where the shaman does most of her work. This is where we store psychic trauma. This field surrounding the body is also impacted by physical assaults to the flesh and bone body, so when we have surgery, or an injury, the energetic body is also impacted. By the same token, we can influence the healing tempo of the physical body by working to heal the energetic body.

Caution: If your dog is pregnant, do not work on the lower three chakras, 1st, 2nd, or 3rd. You can use the pendulum to gauge the pregnancy's health, but do not unwind the lower chakras.

Chakras: the benevolent tornadoes

Eastern philosophy has given us a way to talk about parts of the energetic body. Generally, there are seven

Spirit Dogs

---

bodily areas of the energy field. We call them *chakras* after the Eastern tradition, and we describe them as being funnel-like with their energy spinning in a clockwise fashion when they are functioning correctly. Interestingly, other cultures identify similar fields independent of being aware of the Eastern modality. These are very ancient and intuitive descriptions. Sometimes one culture or another will emphasize different numbers of fields or give more importance to one chakra or another. For example, the Q'ero of Peru speak of the *cosco* which is near the navel on the body as being the seat or center of the spirit, whereas Eastern beliefs generally connect to spirit via the 7th or crown chakra located logically at the top of the head. Coincidentally, however, the *cosco* is the same place as the Chinese medicine "spirit burner" one of the triad of places in the body that hold *chi*. There is a universal and ancient awareness of the presence

Energy Field Basics

---

and importance of energy with regard to the function of the body.

We think of the chakras as having clockwise motion, like a benevolent tornado. Each extends about a foot out from the body, the tip at the body and opened widest farther away. The chakras are counted from 1 to 7 (there are more in some cultures, but they tend to be cosmic in nature and not of the body so we won't worry about them here). Our goal is always to keep the seven chakras spinning clockwise and with equal force. Out of balance chakras may reveal themselves through a variety of responses in the pendulum: by making the pendulum run counterclockwise, or static, or it might shiver and jump. We use the pendulum as a tool to take the pulse of the chakra, much as one would use a thermometer to take the temperature of a feverish child. We're going to use the pendulum as a gauge of the emotional contentment of our dog.

When working with your dog, you will have options: if my dog, Tweed, is lying on his side, I will work along the side that faces up rather than along his spine. I've had dogs roll onto their backs which is great

Spirit Dogs

for a short check, but as you know, dogs don't stay in that position for long. Allow your dog to be comfortable and work with whatever side faces you. You can also place your other hand over the area of the dog's chakra and then read the pendulum, but you must be adept at discerning that you are reading your dog's energy and not interfering with it.

1st Chakra - The Base of the Tail

The 1st chakra is located at the base of the body. On you this would be the perineum between your sexual organs and the anus. On your dog this is at the same place, or if your dog is lying down on his side, it is at the base of the tail. The 1st chakra is his grounding to the Earth and to this lifetime. It is also indicative of his position in the tribe, the pack. A dog happy with his status will have a healthy 1st chakra. A dog with a weak 1st chakra may be uncomfortable with this lifetime or be preparing to move on. A puppy may have a weak 1st chakra simply because he hasn't established his place

Energy Field Basics

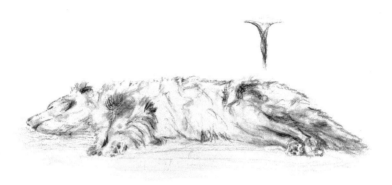

in the pack yet. Keeping in mind that your dog's pack includes you and the other humans and pets in the family, a slow or reversing 1st chakra might mean problems with other pack members. Your dog's basic needs come through at the level of the 1st chakra: hot/cold, hungry, thirsty, afraid. If your dog tucks his tail in fear around other dogs and you check his chakras, probably the 1st chakra will be out of balance, his relationship to his pack needs work. (Unless he's a working border collie, in which case you expect to see a tucked tail!).

Spirit Dogs

2nd *Chakra - The Sexual Center*

The 2nd chakra governs the reproductive organs, even if your dog has been spayed or neutered, the energy is still there! To some degree this chakra is about attitude. Balance is the key word. A dog with a weak 2nd chakra may be meek or might display aggression, either way is out of balance. The 2nd chakra is also about being logical. Before you laugh about your dog being logical, think about it. They understand logic. They know how to get your attention, for food, for love, to be taken on a walk. They know one action leads to another, even if they choose to ignore the results. And they understand fearlessness. Even the smallest dog knows how to be fearless. The trick is to be fearless without being

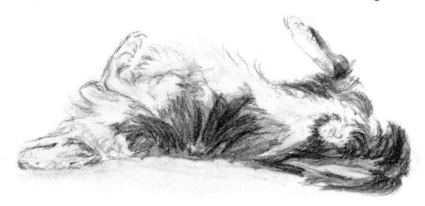

Energy Field Basics

aggressive: *to be beyond fear is a balanced 2nd chakra.* Dogs who bite first and ask questions later need their 2nd chakras brought into balance. In addition, every dog that has undergone reproductive surgery should have their chakras retuned afterwards.

To check this chakra you can access it through the spine parallel to the sex organs or, if they are on their backs for a tummy rub, directly over the area. Because we are all responsible dog owners and have had our dogs spayed or neutered, this chakra can be the first one to show problems. All dogs will be in need of energetic repair following surgery. Conflicts can arise between the Alpha male and his nest mates, everyone's idea of who's important will need refining, soothing.

3rd Chakra - The Solar Plexus

The 3rd chakra centers on the concept of gut instincts, and lies just below the sternum/ribcage juncture. It's that belly we were just rubbing. Dogs with an out of whack 3rd chakra might run away at every opportunity because they think they belong someplace else. Or, similar to the 1st chakra identity, an unbalanced 3rd might come from not knowing their place in the pack so they don't trust their own first instincts. They stand their ground when they shouldn't, nip when they should be enjoying a pat, or refuse to get along with other household members. It's the same for humans, if we don't trust our gut instincts we don't trust each other.

4th Chakra - The Heart

Your dog's heart is, well...it's huge, right? Who loves you more than your dog? No one. The dog's heart chakra is their emotional temperature gauge. They want nothing more than your love and attention (and maybe some more food). Dogs who worry about getting that attention can have unbalanced 4th chakras. Rescue dogs who have been left by previous owners who died or found themselves unable to care for their beloved pets

Energy Field Basics

---

will suffer in their 4th chakras. Matching your 4th chakra to your dog's 4th chakra will tune you into each other. If you're planning to adopt a puppy, spend time with it while it is still in the nursing pen with its mother, matching your heart chakras so it will recognize you and feel your love right from the trip home. Broken-hearted dogs can be very difficult to cure. Working in the energy of the heart chakra is essential to revitalizing a dog that has suffered sadness.

We also use the 4th chakra in conjunction with the 1st chakra to decouple the *fight or flight* response, an essential technique for any dog who has suffered trauma whether it is accidental injury, surgery, a fight with another dog, or abuse. We'll learn how to do this essential work in a later chapter.

5th Chakra -The Throat

Is your dog a barker? Maybe he's trying to tell you something. Dogs who have resorted to constant barking as their means of communication could use

Spirit Dogs

some throat chakra work. The 5th chakra centered on the throat, is our communication switchboard. If your dog's 5th chakra were taxed we would want to know why, which probably will lead to another chakra as well. The 5th chakra messed up is the barking dog. The next chakra that also shows as off balance will indicate the cause. Retuning both chakras so that they work at even cadence with each other will help.

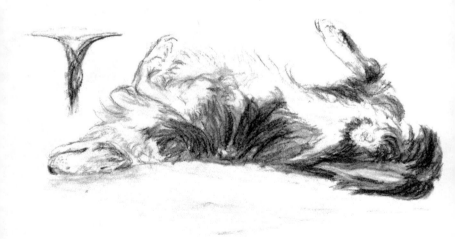

Energy Field Basics

6th Chakra - The Third Eye

The 3rd chakra rules the gut instincts, the 6th is your dog's clairvoyant sense. The 6th chakra is located on the forehead right where it always wrinkles up when your dog is confused by what you're doing.

All dogs have a sixth sense, some highly developed intuitive response that we can't name, but we sure can see it when it happens. We want the dog who knows when there is trouble, who smells it, senses it, and protects us. We want the 6th chakra "Lassie" moment: we don't know how the dog knew Timmy fell down the well, but we're really glad he's here making us check that well. This is the 6th chakra work, it's not gut instinct, it's something from a higher plane. We want this chakra to run in balance with the others. This is the dog's energetic operating system center. Often, our actions alone can control the balance of this chakra. If we ignore our dog when he tries to tell us something, tries to lead us to see something important, we tamp down the 6th chakra. Eventually, the dog will quit trying to give you a heads up when you need one. A rub on

Spirit Dogs

---

the nose, a scratch on the forehead and we're saying "good dog" for using his clairvoyant instincts.

7th Chakra - The Crown

The last of the body chakras is the 7th, the connection to *spirit*. This is the avenue through which your dog came into being and how he will leave when he's ready. This is the life force from wherever it is that all dogs come. This is the connection to god in all forms. We want to see a balance among all the chakras but particularly we want the 7th connection to Spirit to be equal to the 1st connection to Earth. This is a dog who is alive and well. Old or ailing dogs that are readying themselves to die will show a weak or erratic 7th chakra.

We will learn in our final chapter how to assist in making the final voyage a gentle and clear one by working on releasing the chakras, concluding with the 7th. ***Read through all of the steps of the process before you begin working with your own dog.***

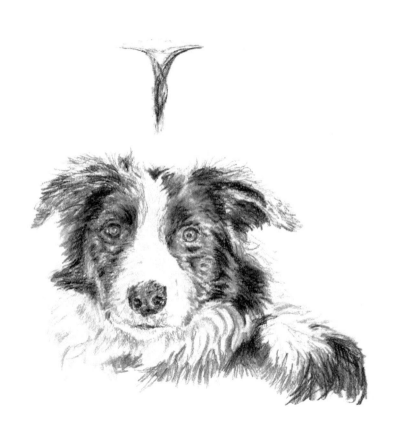

Chapter 3

The Pendulum

A shaman uses his senses to track. Whether it's a Siberian shaman looking for wild game or an Amazonian shaman searching the jungle for natural medicine or checking his community for illness, a trained shaman can look at what he is inquiring about and *see* the energy without any tools other than his mind and eyes. In the folk language of ancient Briton and Ireland, he has "the sight." Through a process of opening up the capability of the third eye, 6th chakra, the trained shaman has access to extra senses with which to track for illness and disturbance. Clairvoyance, clairessence, clairsentience, these are all expansions of our normal senses that any of us, with training and dedication, can use. The pendulum just makes the work easier. It's an

The Pendulum

extension of your non-thinking brain. I know a shaman who doesn't use a pendulum, but he uses the smoke trail from an incense stick and watches the smoke for direction, strength, and pattern. We're going to use a pendulum. (See Appendices for additional information.)

Let's get started. There is only one tool you need to do this work: a pendulum. The pendulum can be anything: a necklace or a dedicated purchased pendulum—something fancy with a pointed crystal on the end—it doesn't matter. What matters is that the pendulum itself is evenly weighted and of sufficient weight to move freely. It should have a chain long enough, perhaps a 20" chain, and slippery enough not to impede the movement of the pendulum. Even though a charm on the end of a leather cord will work, it won't be as easy to use as a chain. If you have a necklace on, take it off (or borrow it from your girlfriend), fold the chain across your palm and dangle about 8 inches of chain and the pendant charm at the end. Hold still. This is pretty much the position. Now let's back up a minute. Take a look at the pendant you've decided to use. Is it evenly weighted front and back? Balanced? The weight

Spirit Dogs

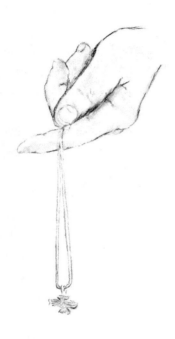

of a penny would be perfect. I have a couple of necklaces with charms that are the same on both sides—equal weight, that's what we're after. The next thing I personally think is important is that the pendulum be energetically aligned with you. If you bought it new, you need to make it your own. You can do this by cupping the pendulum in your hands and blowing your breath over it. If it's wearable—and usually it is, put it on and wear it for a few days with intention: "this is my pendulum." If you aren't into jewelry, put it in your pocket and now and then give it some attention.

The Pendulum

Practice

To start, we don't need the dog. Practice holding the pendulum lightly, without intentionally moving it (because we all have a heartbeat, there will be some movement of your hand, you can't help it—just don't deliberately spin it). Hold it over the floor. Then hold it over your other hand, palm up. Did anything different happen? Now hold it over water. Yes! You are dowsing! Last fall my husband did some yard work. The dogs had managed to uncover the septic tank lid and dug a bunch of holes he had to fill in. But he was sure there was a second septic lid. He asked me to help. I used the pendulum to track what I was looking for, in the same way that a dowser uses dowsing rods to find water. Using the pendulum in this way is primarily about setting an intention: to find water, or a lost item, whatever you place in your consciousness as the connection between yourself and the pendulum (or dowsing rod). Focused intention is a powerful tool. I walked the area near the first tank, and right away found where I thought the lid would be based on the wild, and I mean

Spirit Dogs

wild, gyrations of my pendulum. "Oh no," he said. "It's not there, that's downhill. Look uphill." OK, so I looked uphill. Nothing. Meanwhile, he was busy digging test holes uphill (why didn't he let the dogs do that?) with no results. I went back across the area I'd been before. Wild spinning, in fact, I've never seen my pendulum react so strongly. I started kicking dirt with my foot. "Come on, humor me," I said. And there it was, downhill, right where the pendulum said it would be. I think the pendulum reacted so strongly because the septic tank was full of water, and water dowsing is a classic and easy use of this technique.

Practice with your pendulum, get to know what it knows, how it likes to express itself. Clockwise is good, counterclockwise is bad, static pulsing is worrying, or sometimes it just means energy is moving—as if the pendulum is thinking. I don't usually see diagonal movements with mine, but people are different. You have to learn how to use your own pendulum and establish firmly what it means to you when it acts in different ways, but for now, keep it simple. It may take time for the pendulum to begin to move. You may

The Pendulum

want to stop it with your other hand to a dead stop before starting a new test over a new chakra. Eventually you will develop a smooth motion where the pendulum will stop on its own as you move from one chakra to the other. Try not to encourage the pendulum to move, it's amazing how hard it is to truly stay still, but the reward of letting the pendulum move on its own is that you will have more confidence in the result. I know master shaman who look like they are pushing the pendulum, and it seems to work for them, but we're not asking to be master shaman, we're just learning how to use the best tool for this work.

Once you have made the pendulum your own, here is the step by step process for checking your dog's chakras:

Position

If you can get your dog to lie down and stay put and still be relaxed then apparently you don't have a border collie. I try to wait until my dog is already in a good position and is calm, even sleeping, before I pull out my pendulum. As long as they are calm you can pretty much check their chakras no matter what position they are in, but obviously lying out straight is easiest.

Opening sacred space

By *sacred* I mean that we are focusing our own consciousness within a specific ritual process in order to heighten our connection or attention to the subject, in this case, our dog. *Sacred* and *ritual* are universal words that do not define and are not the provenance of any particular organized religion. They refer to a way of bringing our focus, our actions, our whole being into mindful attention. By performing a ritual we acknowledge our intent to right action, our willingness to embrace the harnessed power of the process. The shaman always works for the good of the community, positive power results from embracing the ritual sacred landscape. Really what we are asking for here is mindful attention in the classic Buddhist sense. The

The Pendulum

more we can bring our whole energetic being to focus on our dog, the more successful we will be at helping him. I'm reminded of Albert Einstein's quip: "If you can drive safely while kissing a girl, you are simply not giving the kiss the attention it deserves." The creation of ritual sacred space is a simple process of focus, a way to inform the body that what we are going to do next is important and powerful.

We want to envelop our dog in an invisible security blanket of our calm and loving energy. There's a nice yoga mudra you can use where you reach your arms up over your head with palms together in prayer pose, and then lean forward as if laying an invisible blanket across your dog. You've created a shared energetic realm between yourself and your dog. It is a ritual, and its action takes you from regular day-to-day stuff into the realm of the spiritual. You and your dog are safe.

The Pendulum

Blow on your pendulum to clear it of any previous energy. If your dog is awake and curious, let him smell the pendulum. Slide the chain across your palm and let the pendulum dangle. Relax. Don't deliberately move the pendulum but you'll see that it's pretty impossible to hold completely still, don't worry: the pendulum will do what it will do regardless. Hold it about 5 inches above your dog's body directly above the 1st chakra. Don't be surprised if it takes a moment or two for the pendulum to begin the first time you read it. Be patient. Often you will see the pendulum jump or jiggle as it connects to the energy. This is good.

Don't be surprised if your dog notices. He can feel you in his energy field. Reassure him, but if he gets too agitated, play with him and resume the pendulum later, or even another day.

Check each chakra from 1st to 7th. Allow the pendulum to reset between each one. Observe the seven reactions of the pendulum but check all 7 chakras

The Pendulum

before you decide how to proceed with the healing process.

Make notes on how the dog and the pendulum reacted. Were the chakras all about equal in strength of motion—were they all eliciting a clockwise response at about the same rate?

If yes, excellent. Then you're done for the day. Remove your protective energy from over your dog by reversing the motion of lifting the invisible safety blanket and bringing it back to your own head, heart, and lap. Blow on your pendulum to clear it.

But if you found one or more chakras out of balance, move on to the next chapter to learn where healing begins.

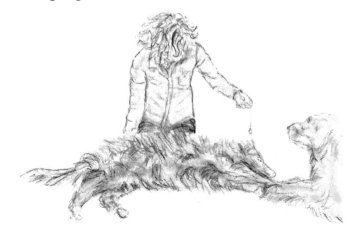

Chapter 4

Tuning the Out of Balance Chakra

I was taught that if there is more than one chakra out of balance, treat the lowest number first because often that will reset the others as well. So, for example, if the 1st and 3rd chakras are spinning counterclockwise, treat the 1st chakra first. However, gauge your dog. How much will he sit still for? Is there an obvious issue? Remember about my dog with the epilepsy? If, following a seizure, his 3rd, 6th, and 7th chakras were out of balance I wouldn't bother right away with the 3rd because I'd know where the problem was. His 3rd chakra might be out because he was confused and unsure of what just happened, but the issue rests with the brain, the 6th chakra. Use your own instincts! Since we can't be sure how long you'll have this compliant

Tuning the Out of Balance Chakra

dog in front of you, work on the chakra that appears to need it the most. Then check and recheck with your pendulum. Often, other chakras will come into line on their own.

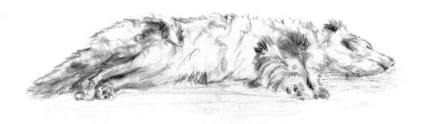

Process

To clear a blocked, erratic, or backed up chakra we use our hand and with a wave (imagine Queen Elizabeth only round and round upside-down), fingers pointing down, unwind the chakra. Remember that the chakra is a funnel about 8 inches high. Unwind it as if you are tracing the outside of the funnel, creating a counter-

Spirit Dogs

clockwise tornado as you lift your hand from near the dog to higher up.

Now that the chakra is unwound hold your hand, palm down, above the chakra and fill the area with gentleness and healing, moving softly over the chakra area. Sometimes people think of this as filling it with sunlight. Pour all your love into the chakra. Then very slowly and gently, rewind the chakra with your hand in clockwise motion. Recheck the chakras with your pendulum. Repeat this with the other unbalanced chakra points. Recheck all chakras with your pendulum one last time. Never leave a chakra unwound. I like to finish with a quick clockwise tune up of all seven chakras one final time before closing the session. When you have finished, all seven chakras should stimulate the pendulum to a clockwise motion of about the same amount.

Tuning the Out of Balance Chakra

Deeper work: injury, illness, surgery

Dogs who have just suffered injury, illness, or surgery will need to have their energy field "repaired." Think of the energy field as a sleeping bag with your dog in it. Repairing it zips it back up. We do this by working well above the area that was injured, using our hand without touching the dog, by scooping out infection, and then patting and soothing the energy back into place. Do this with a sleeping or very calm dog, and with great care: do not disturb the dog. Once you've practiced, you can do this just by thinking over your dog with focused mindfulness.

Quick Guide

Basic Checkup
- open a safe energy space from yourself to your dog
- check chakras from 1 to 7 with pendulum
- note out of balance chakra(s) work from lowest # up
- unwind (counterclockwise) one chakra at a time with your hand
- bring in love and light, sun, and healing
- rewind (clockwise) chakra and retest with pendulum
- repeat with other unbalanced chakras
- check with pendulum, rewind all clockwise one last time
- remove your shared energy safety "blanket"

Chapter 5

Decoupling Fight or Flight

I first practiced this on my cousin's Siberian husky. He was a two year old dog when they adopted him from a shelter. While all huskies have reputations for running—it is, after all, what they were bred for—Kenai was a specialist. I thought part of the problem was that he was confused about who he belonged to. To start, I checked his chakras and found that his 1st and 3rd chakras were

Spirit Dogs

---

in counterclockwise motion: in other words, he didn't know where his tribe was, and he didn't trust his gut instinct. He was a loving amenable dog in all other ways, but he showed his insecurity by some nervous traits besides taking off: he would suck on his flank when insecure. I worked with him several times over the years. Each time I would make sure to decouple the flight or fight instinct because in any stressful situation, that is the first response. He settled in quickly and displayed his natural insecurities less and less as he grew completely happy with his new home. Here's how to do it.

There are two aspects to Decoupling Fight or Flight. The first use of this process is for general stability in your dog. If your dog has suddenly experienced trauma, skip the preliminary chakra cleansing process and go right to holding the heart and 2nd chakra as described below. Then once the dog calms down, you can return to a regular check and cleanse of all chakras. Read through the process below to see the details.

Decoupling Fight or Flight

Process: Decoupling Fight or Flight— Non-Emergency method

All rescued dogs will need their fight or flight response decoupled, and careful regulation of their heart chakras is always needed.

Begin by opening your energy field over your dog just as described earlier in the pendulum tracking instructions. Check your dog's chakras with the pendulum and tune them as they present themselves just as you've already learned to do.

Next—and this will work best with a very calm or sleeping dog but do your best, if the dog is in fight or flight he probably won't be all that calm—place your palms on your dog at the 2nd chakra. If you can, have them underneath the dog, between the dog and the ground. Relax your hands. If your dog won't allow that, place your palms on top of the dog's body just before the leg/flank begins. Gently. Softly talk to your dog in a reassuring voice. To a human, we would say something like "it's all right, my love." To your dog, you might

Spirit Dogs

say, "good dog, sweet dog." It's all about your voice. Try to imagine connecting your dog's 2nd chakra to the earth through your hands, a single line of belonging, of grounding. Hold this position for a minute or two. Then move one palm up to the heart chakra. See if you can feel your dog's heartbeat. A small dog who is lying in your lap will probably allow you to hold it with one hand beneath the 2nd and one hand beneath the heart; a bigger dog might not want your hands underneath, do what works. Feel the heartbeat connect with your heartbeat and with the heartbeat of the Earth. When you sense that the connection is made you can gently remove your hands. Leave sleeping dogs lie, as they say. Remove your energy blanket and bring it back into your own heart.

Decoupling fight or flight response is essential after trauma, surgery, adoption, or for any dog that has lost his owner. It resets the defensive system but also resets the immune response making for a healthier dog. Miraculously, you'll find as you decouple your dog's defensive response mechanism your own will decouple as well! This is because, in our hectic worlds

Decoupling Fight or Flight

it is too often the case that we are tossed into a fight or flight reactive state. Do this process on your dog every time you check his energetic health.

Process: Decoupling Fight or Flight—Emergency Process

A dog who is injured, terrified, or had any sort of sudden trauma or shock whether emotional or physical needs help immediately. If your dog will let you cradle it, or hold it firmly, skip the chakra check portion of the previous instructions and follow the directions for decoupling just as described previously:

Place your palms on your dog at the 2nd chakra. If you can, have them underneath the dog, between the dog and the ground. Relax your hands. If your dog won't allow that, place your palms on top of the dog's body just before the leg/flank begins. Gently. Softly talk to your dog in a reassuring voice. To a human, we would say something like "it's all right, my love." To your dog, you might say, "good dog, sweet dog." It's all

Spirit Dogs

about your voice. Try to imagine connecting your dog's 2nd chakra to the earth through your hands, a single line of belonging, of grounding. Hold this position for a minute or two. Then move one palm up to the heart chakra. See if you can feel your dog's heartbeat. Feel your dog's heartbeat connect with your heartbeat and with the heartbeat of the Earth. Connecting your dog with the Mother. Imagine a tether connecting your dog's heart down into the depths of the earth. When you sense that the connection is made you can gently remove your hands.

When I've needed to work with a dog in crisis mode, I find it helpful to give an alcohol-free version of Bach Flower therapy Rescue Remedy for animals. A few drops in water.

Once you have decoupled fight or flight, you can check the dog's chakras and reset them as needed.

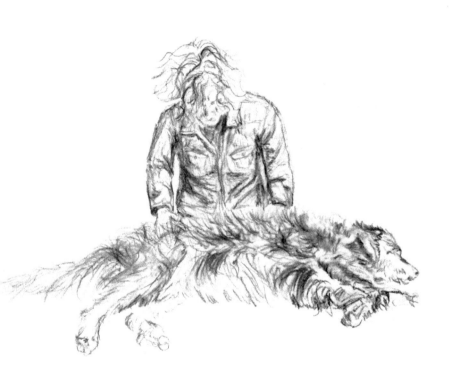

Chapter 6

Saying Goodbye

This is the hardest work we will ever do, saying goodbye and letting our loved ones, whether they be human or canine or feline, die. Dying consciously is a very specialized and carefully practiced shamanic art. It may well be the most powerful and spiritual ritual act we engage, and it must be approached seriously. The essence of it, though, has to do with opening up and releasing the chakras; and this is something you can do yourself with your dog. If you are faced with having your dog euthanized, whether your dog has died suddenly and traumatically, or peacefully and naturally, you can spend your final moments with your dog creating a quiet and safe pathway for his spirit. Not only will it make dying calmer and easier for your

Saying Goodbye

dog, it will give you a way to feel less helpless and process your grief in a meaningful way. Any time we practice ritual and create ceremony we are honoring the energy of the sacred mysteries.

Caution: This is powerful work. It should only be undertaken at the time of death or just afterwards.

As with every other use of this chakra-tending energy medicine, the first thing to do is to use the pendulum to check your dog's chakras. The responses of the chakras will tell you a lot about whether your dog is ready to leave this lifetime. Kenai was suffering with a spinal issue that was giving him pain. It seemed as though he should have been gathering himself to approach death, and yet, over several months when I would check his chakras, he still seemed quite present in this life and not at all ready. His crown chakra was strong, so his exit strategy was positive and in place but he seemed to remain content with life in spite of the pain. Eventually, he began to show less power in his lower, earthly chakras, and more movement

Spirit Dogs

upward into the gateway of the crown. At that point we knew he was nearly ready. Always check your dog's chakras: allow them to guide your decisions as to how to proceed. Let it be his decision.

When it is time, you will know it. Your dog is suffering and unsure. He doesn't want to leave you; you don't want him to leave. This is such a difficult moment. You and your veterinary advisors have agreed about what's best for his welfare. You already know to reassure your dog that it's OK to go, that you love him, that you'll see him again. But it is time. He may already have died, or be at the very edge just before euthanizing. You may be lucky enough to be at home with your dog or you may have traveled to the safety of your vet's office with family gathered around. When you are certain that he is ready, you may begin. Or you may choose to perform this ritual after your dog has been euthanized, which works just as well, and may be easier if the dog is at all agitated. As difficult as it may seem, I speak from experience when I say that it will be better for your dog and for you to be present and in a ceremonial, ritual state of sacredness at his death. Honoring your bond one last time.

You have already checked your dog's chakras and made the decisions and arrangements that will allow for his passing. Make him comfortable. Take as long as you need to bring your own energy into a sense of ritual. When Fionn died I laid him on one of my Q'ero Peruvian blankets, opened my medicine bundle, and arranged my sacred stones around and on his body. I lit incense and candles and sat with him for a while, remembering our time together, and yes, weeping with sadness at his parting. When it was time, I knew it. The energy in the room shifted. It was time to release him.

Process

Essentially, we are reversing the process of chakra tuning, opening up each chakra, beginning with the 1st and working slowly toward the 7th with plenty of time at each one to allow the transition to begin. With the

Spirit Dogs

release of the 7th and final chakra, the body, energetic and corporeal, will be ready to go.

To begin: as always, envelop your dog in ritual sacred space. Now, beginning with the base, the 1st chakra, and using your hand about 6 inches above his body, unwind the chakra in a counterclockwise motion. Then unwind the heart chakra. Take your time, do this work gently. This is a sacred ceremony. You might have a special cloth picked out, a ritual blanket that will go with your dog. No matter where you are, whether you are at home, at the veterinary hospital, wherever, make it sacred. This is about saying goodbye, about honoring, and grieving. Move from the first open chakra to the heart, then to the 2nd chakra, and back to the heart. And then on to the 3rd and back to the heart. You are making graceful spirals of the exiting energy. In between, speak to your dog, talk about your life together. We do this with our human family when they are preparing to pass on, reconciling our lives together. It allows us, the living, to move on and equips the dead to make the passage. Go through all of the chakras, always returning to the heart. The 7th chakra

Saying Goodbye

is the moment when the energetic body takes over from the physical and orchestrates the transformation to the otherworld. Spirit takes charge. Now your dog can move peacefully into the otherworld. Remove the ritual sacred space, bringing your own energy back into your heart.

A note about afterwards: it is generally held among shaman that we should allow the body at least a day to release the spirit before cremation.

Final Words

Dogs are incredibly intuitive, more intuitive than we are. That sixth sense, whatever it is, is already very well established in our canine friends. I suppose the heightened development of their senses, such as hearing and smell, are part of their survival mechanism over many, many generations since the prehistoric times when they were wild wolves. Surely their intuitive sense belongs in this category. Often, we find dogs choose us, rather than the other way around. We have a lot to learn from our pets, about loyalty, love, and coping strategies for difficult times.

Even dogs that have been abused and seem to be beyond our reach have, with care, the ability to be happy, healthy companions. It is possible that the best thing we can do for them is try to be tuned into their energy 100% of the time. This book is for the times

Final Words

when we aren't sure, when we suddenly look at our dog and think, "Hmmm, wonder what's up with Rowdy. He looks worried, or tired, or stressed (you fill in the blank). I wonder why." Rowdy might be an aptly named 80 lb. rescued dog living the high life with his litter mate, an 80 lbs. "don't worry, be happy" dog, safe and loved in Dallas right now with their 110 lb. human, but that doesn't mean there aren't days when he's not at his loyal best. Working through the simple techniques of this book, Rowdy's "mom" can get solid clues about what otherwise might be no more than a mystery locked deep in his canine psyche. This simple tracking technique gives you an edge. It's not a replacement for good veterinary care, a healthy diet, and lots of exercise. But this method of tracking the emotional temperature of your pet unlocks an area of understanding your dog that isn't covered by vets, diet, or exercise. Most of the time, dogs are trying very hard to communicate with us. Tap into your own inner shaman and learn to hear them better. And now, it appears my two guys are saying it's time to stop typing and play ball.

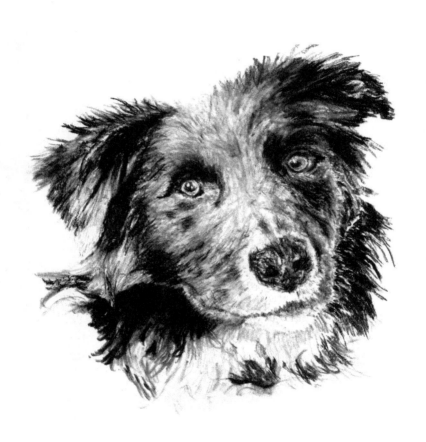

Appendices

What about cats, horses, & absentee animals?

All of these techniques can be applied to both cats and horses but obviously with some changes in how to approach the animal. Working with cats is interesting because it has been my experience that cats are very intuitive about energy. I've often had acupuncture or massage treatments at home and couldn't keep my cat off the massage table. During one acupuncture session the cat was insistent enough that my acupuncturist finally asked me what was up with my cat, and then she inserted some needles to help with some pain the cat chronically experienced, and he was fine. The primary challenge with working on cats is that they think the pendulum is a toy for them to bat and snag with their claws. It's better to catch the cat sleeping.

Appendices

Horses are such sentient beings, deeply deeply aware, empathic, and equipped with such huge hearts. I've never owned a horse, but if I were to work on a horse energetically I would work on the tracking while doing some basic grooming for to start. Use your hand as a connect so that the pendulum isn't a distraction or startles the horse. A lot can be learned simply by using the pendulum over the 6th chakra. Hold your palm above the eyes where you would normally give your horse a scratch or pat and use the pendulum in your other hand, away from the horse. You can follow the chakras down the back of the horse, or up from the rear along the back, the placement of the chakras won't change, and how you get to the horse to use the pendulum will depend on you and the horse but you can even sit on the horse and do it from that position.

Checking on an animal when you are not with them is a great thing to do. It takes mindfulness skills but with practice you will be able to track your pet from a distance and be confident in your results. Set a ritual space as if your pet were there lying in front of you. The ritual intensity of this approach is very important.

Spirit Dogs

The more fully focused you are the clearer the picture will be and the more confident you can be that you are seeing the energy results correctly. I've done this with cats that have wandered off. In fact, finding pets who are lost is a great use of this remote viewing method. In this case, once you have set the ritual space, you can visualize your pet, throw out a line to it, an energy line, and then reel them in. It works. For a basic tracking or check-in with your pet (and by that I mean you will be letting your pet know you are thinking about him) set the ritual space, visualize your pet in front of you, soften your gaze like you do in yoga, and use the pendulum to check the chakras. Send your pet energy and love, give the chakras a clockwise tune up, and a calming blanket of good energy. Close the ritual space. I always blow on my pendulum at the end of any session to clear it and to make it ready to use the next time.

Making Your Own Pendulum

Perhaps the best way to work with a pendulum at peak efficiency is to have one that is truly your own, one that is saturated with your energy, if you will. The most complete way to do this is to build your own. One of my favorite, and most powerful pendulum pieces was made for me by my shaman friend and amazing jewelry maker, Jillian Vogtli. She used bead wire and a variety of stones to create the perfect pendulum: it has balance, and sufficient weight, and it is filled with the love we have for each other in our friendship, as well as the particular energetic essential meanings of the stones she chose to use which include labradorite, known as the shaman's stone, sleeping beauty turquoise, onyx, and amber. I added to that base my grandfather's dog tag from WWI. The result is a beautiful necklace that has serious energetic power. I also have a plain silver

Spirit Dogs

chain with a round pointed quartz on the end, a standard "pendulum" purchased at a bead store. You can buy pendulums in all sorts of styles with simple quartz crystals on the ends. There is a lot of information available about the power of crystals– their ability to pull in and hold energy. This power makes a quartz crystal a very good choice for a first pendulum. Find a piece that looks clean, meaning not "dirty" with non quartz streaks inside, and is free of cracks and surface flaws. Completely clear faceted pieces of quartz are hard to find and it isn't necessary but of course, clear pieces are considered stronger. For more information about crystals look for Kirby Seid crystals and the work of Marcel Vogel online.

I've made several pendulums for myself and really enjoyed choosing the charms and assembling the piece. There's something about creating your own that really helps develop the energetic connection. To make your own piece, use bead wire and regular beading techniques, or use a chain and find a simple charm that will be your designated tool. It doesn't have to be fancy, but it is a very good idea for your first pendulum

Appendices

to be a dedicated working tool, not a random piece of jewelry, at least until you get a good grasp of the process. Once you have finished your piece, clean the energy by blowing your breath over it, place it on your altar, smug with incense or a candle in any way that signifies ritual importance for you.

While I have several dedicated pendulums, I also commonly use whatever necklace I'm wearing. But before I do that, I always blow my breath over the necklace to cleanse it and bring it into alignment energetically– it's a way of focusing both myself and the pendulum to the moment at hand. With practice some people are able to simply "look" at whatever they want to track, and it is possible to see energy emanate from the body, it rather looks like gasoline fumes to me. There are shamanic rites and rituals dedicated to preparing the shaman to see in this way, and usually takes practice to perfect in the same way that meditation takes practice to learn how to work with consciousness to reach the goal of mindfulness.

Log Book

I've always kept a diary or medical log for my dogs but this habit intensified with Tweed who has tried many various medication combinations and needed to have his reactions cataloged. When training to do shamanic energy work we kept written records of our training sessions and wrote up formal reports. For those of us planning to establish formal practices in energy medicine this was excellent training of habit for the future. The following pages are for your notes. Similarities in, for example, stressful times of year, or changes in environment or even the seasons will show up with regular checks and good note taking!

Develop your own pattern. Some ideas might be to give chakra pendulum checks a rating, say, one to four stars, a directional indication, and a strength. For example: Heart chakra 3* strong clockwise. Even if

Appendices

a chakra is running in balance, it's good to note how strongly and how well in relation to the others which you can tell by the * rating. If the 3rd chakra is 2* and the 6th is 4* there is an imbalance even if the pendulum doesn't indicate a counterclockwise direction. The optimum is a dog with all seven chakras at 4* clockwise. You may use the following pages, copy them, or create your own.

Date _____ *Record of Session with* _____
Description of issue/symptoms: _____
_____
_____
_____

Chakra assessment/* rating and direction:

1/   2/   3/   4/

5/   6/   7/

Work done: _____
_____
_____
_____

Conclusion: _____
_____
_____
_____

Follow-up: _____
_____
_____
_____

Veterinary visit summary: _____
_____
_____
_____

Date _____ Record of Session with _____
Description of issue/symptoms: _____
_____
_____
_____

Chakra assessment/* rating and direction:

1/   2/   3/   4/

5/   6/   7/

Work done: _____
_____
_____
_____

Conclusion: _____
_____
_____
_____

Follow-up: _____
_____
_____
_____

Veterinary visit summary: _____
_____
_____
_____

Author Jane Galer holds a BA in philosophy, an MA in material culture studies, and a certificate in museum curation for archaeologists. She trained as a shaman in the lineage of the Q'ero of Peru. Her work includes *Becoming Hummingbird: Charting Your Life Journey the Shaman's Way*, *The Navigator's Wife*, a novel, and mostly recently the poetry collection, *Outskirts* (2016). She is currently at work on *The Painted People: The Celtic Shaman's Lineage*. Jane lives in northern California with her husband, Gene, and border collies, Tweed and Cavendish.

Illustrator Kim Englishbee resides in Texas where she continues her love affair with creative arts and her husband Ron.

About the Dogs

Cavendish and Tweed are pure bred border collies from a Scottish bloodline. They are our hearts, litter mates yet as different as could be. Four years ago, thinking I might have only one more puppy training siege in me, Gene and I decided on these two from a local, respected, small breeder who had also been the source of our previous two lovely border collies. We picked them out as wiggling three week old puppies and visited them often until they were old enough to come home with us. We live on a ten-acre tract of forest, and the dogs have free range, never restricted in their adventures. I grew up with cats, not dogs, but have come to find the companionship of dogs sustaining and irreplaceable in ways so different to our feline friends.

Blue and Rowdy were adopted by Kathie and Dave through a local Australian Shepherd Rescue in the Dallas/Ft Worth area when they were just turning one. The brothers were surrendered by their owners to a rural shelter when they had lost their home. Blue is an adorable big lug of a dog—Aussie and Bernese Mountain Dog mix. He loves people, sleeping, and hunting frogs and lizards in his own backyard. His brother, Rowdy, is Aussie and Golden Retriever mix (yes, you can have multiple fathers in the same litter!). Rowdy is true to both of his parents in that he is always at your heels and as loyal as they come. He loves to "help" around the house—whatever Kathie does, he is always there to lend a helping paw. Kathie and Dave only planned to get one dog. After they met the two dogs they agreed to count to 3 and say out loud which one they should take home...one said black and one said brown. So, they compromised and took both. It's five years later, and they are so glad they were able to rescue them both. The dogs love each other and oftentimes can be seen sleeping or lying down in the exact same position. Where one is, the other is only a few steps away. As it should be.

Diane and Jerry rescued Kenai, a two and a half year-old Siberian Husky. He and several litter mates were also given up by a family affected by economic hardship. The Bay Area (San Francisco) Siberian Husky Club's rescue and referral program quickly found homes for all the litter mates. A runner by nature, Kenai would bolt at any opportunity during the early years of adoption. Eventually, he adjusted to his new environment and traded in bolting (and getting lost) for the occassional meander around the neighborhood (and finding his way back home). A handsome black and white Husky with blue eyes and the ability to smile, he was gentle and loving throughout his long, fifteen and a half year life.

Acknowledgments

My trio of talented and amazing cousins: Diane Reynolds, Kim Englishbee, and Kathie Britton have made this book possible. I could not have done it without them. Kathie edited the manuscript along the way, and she and her wonderful dogs were models and "guinea pigs" for the illustrations. Kim drew the perfect illustrations. Diane is my partner in producing these books, and as always, all this is simply not possible without her support, expertise, and project manager and designer acumen.

Thanks also to Christine Paul Costello for her friendship, and her initial trust in me, to Jon Rasmussen for insisting on formal shamanic training and helping me follow this path. Karen Taylor Bryan and Kristi Matson Hahn for their friendship. And, to the dogs: Sam, Ciara, Fionn, Tweed and Cavendish, Rowdy and

Blue, and Kenai. You taught me so much, and fill my heart.

Finally, books don't happen without a support system that includes an understanding, patient, and generous family. I am always grateful that I married the perfect person.

Jane's Dog Biscotti

There is anecdotal evidence that gluten may cause an increase in epilesy in dogs so we make gluten free biscotti. If this isn't a concern, you can use standard baking mix instead. Makes 40-45 3-inch biscotti.

2 packages Bob's Red Mill Gluten Free Biscuit & Baking Mix
1 package organic bacon
4 T organic peanut butter
1 qt. organic beef broth
2 cups grated cheddar cheese

Optional:
2 T molasses (iron rich)
1/2 cup organic pure pumpkin (pumpkin is for dogs with digestive upset, diarrhea)

Preheat oven to 400°F. Cover two cookie sheets with parchment paper.

In a large bowl mix the gluten free flour with the cheese. Add peanut butter and rub in until pebbly, or cut in with a pastry blender or two knives.

Cut the bacon into ½ inch pieces and fry until crispy. Do not drain. Pour hot grease and bacon into the dry ingredients. Add the beef broth and stir with a large spoon. Add water as necessary to make the dough hold together. Without gluten, the dough will be shaggy until there is enough water.

Turn the dough onto a floured surface and mold with your hands until it holds together. Pat into a large rectangle, evening out the sides, and roll with a rolling pin until the dough is 1–1½ inches thick and even.

Have flour nearby to keep the cookie cutter from sticking. Cut the dough into dog bone shape biscuits and place on cookie sheet. Reshape scraps and roll out, repeating until all dough has been cut into shape.

Bake for 35 minutes or until golden brown. If you have a convection oven, bake with convection ON. When the biscuits are golden brown, turn the heat off but leave the convection fan on, if you can, with the biscuits still in the oven. This will dry out the biscuits into biscotti.

When the biscotti are thoroughly dry and cool, place a one week's supply in a container for hard treats. Divide the remaining biscotti into 1 week servings, place in zip lock freezer bags, and freeze.

CPSIA information can be obtained
at www.ICGtesting.com
Printed in the USA
BVHW090625091019
560603BV00004B/53/P